THE PREVENTION OF CONGENITAL MALFORMATIONS DEFECTS AND DISEASES BY THE MEDICINAL AND NUTRITIONAL TREATMENT OF THE MOTHER DURING PREGNANCY.

THE PREVENTION OF CONGENITAL MALFORMATIONS DEFECTS AND DISEASES BY THE MEDICINAL AND NUTRITIONAL TREATMENT OF THE MOTHER DURING PREGNANCY.

BY

J.C. BURNETT, M.D., LONDON.

EDITOR HOMOEO PATHIC WORLD

KALPAZ

ISBN: 978-93-5128-746-9(PB)

First Published in1881
Indian Reprint in 2017

Published by

Kalpaz Publications
C-30, Satyawati Nagar,
Delhi – 110052
E-mail: kalpaz@hotmail.com
Website: kalpazpublications.com
Ph.: +91-9212142040

PREFACE.

The following pages are compiled to diffuse information upon subjects of the deepest medical and philanthropic interest. The facts here given throw light upon subjects of great maternal anxiety. To prevent disease is the highest development of the medical art. To prevent malformations and physical defects in the coming generation is an achievement that should arrest the attention of the civilized world. " To do good and to communicate forget not."

To further the study of this important topic I would adopt the words of Dr. Burnett: " Feeling that the experience of one individual in this branch of *Preventive Medicine* can count for but very little, I should be glad to receive from my readers any information bearing on the subject, either as regards man or the lower animals."

T. C. D.

THE PREVENTION

OF

CONGENITAL MALFORMATIONS.

Preventive medicine is a bold step. It is about a century since Jenner's attention was called to the fact that vaccination with cowpox would prevent an attack of small-pox, and about the same time Hahnemann evolved the new idea that Belladonna would prevent scarlet fever, as then prevailing. He believed that the remedy that would cure a disease would also prevent the same disease. This fact opened up a wide field for experimentation.

The next most important fact in the line of preventive medicine is given by Gŕauvogl, where medicines were administered to correct

ANTENATAL PHYSIOLOGICAL DEFECTS.

He writes as follows:

A young married pair had, two years previously, lost a child from hydrocephalus acutus; the second, then eight months old, was committed to my charge, when the disease had already reached the convulsive stage; it died after a few days.

It devolved now upon me, as the family physician to solve the problem of protecting the next child from this disease, and thus to remove the conditions under which both times, the development of the fatal disease had been possible, a problem which everybody knows the physiological school is not able to solve.

Both parents were perfectly healthy, and never sick. Both had blonde hair, thin skin, and blue eyes. The husband spare; the wife of a full habit. Hence no positive point of support could be gained from either. The wife, however, had nursed both of the children, but without possessing sufficient nourishment for them, as I learned on inquiry, for she was obliged to give them milk, and sugar-water besides and both children were taken sick when they began to *cut their teeth.*

In hydrocephalus the nutrition of the bones is always deficient, and hence, during the period of dentition, this nutrition must be carried on at the expense of other tissues. But the conditions of this deficient nutrition of the osseous system must have been given long before the period of dentition.

I hence stated to the wife that she must not nurse the next child, and that she must, during her next pregnancy take Sulphur 6th one day, and Calcarea phosphoricum 6th, the next, so that she could not lose a third child by this disease.

Sulphur I wished to exhibit as a nutritive remedy favoring the formation of tissue, while Calcarea phosphoricum was to favor that of the bones.

Five weeks later, the woman informed me that she was again pregnant, and asked me for those remedies.

She was delivered at term, and this child, now five years old, remained healthy, as well as a second, now three years old, which was carried the regular term under this prophylactic treatment.

These are not solitary cases, for I have pursued this method for six years, in all families in which there has even been a hydrocephalic child, and with the same good result.

But where I have taken charge, in other families, of children who had already suffered from hydrocephalus none have died during the last seven years, in which time I have given such children, every morning and evening, a powder of the second trit. of Calcarea phosphoricum; and only such children as I first see in the last stage, receive morning and evening, a few drops of Argentum nittricum 6. and every two hours the powder of Calcarea phosphoricum, and with the best -ults. At the sametime, I have repeatedly convinced my-' that, in such cases, one of these remedies alone affords such relief.

r. G. E. Shipman, Superintendent of the Chicago ndlings' Home, reports that he has proved the value of auvogl's prophylactic treatment in several instances. I · also followed this plan with gratifying success.

ON THE PREVENTION OF HARE-LIP, CLEFT-PALATE, AND OTHER CONGENITAL DEFECTS; AS ALSO OF HEREDITARY DISEASE AND CONSTITUTIONAL TAINTS BY THE MEDICINAL AND NUTRITIONAL TREATMENT OF THE MOTHER DURING PREGNANCY.

[Perhaps the most interesting instance of preventive medicine, to the profession and especially to mothers, is where the medicine was given to prevent congenital malformations. The experience of J. C. Burnett, M. D., of London, as given in a paper read before the British Homœopathic Congress, is especially valuable. It shows that what were supposed to be "marks" are due simply to lack of proper nutrition. The full text of the article is here given:]

Mr. President and Gentlemen:—I take the liberty this morning of calling a little special attention to a subject fraught with considerable interest to us as human beings, as men of science, as biologists, and as practitioners of medicine and family advisers.

Should this paper set you a thinking, and call forth a discussion and an expression of opinion, and also elicit the experience of those grown grey in the service of scientific therapeutics, I shall learn much therefrom.

I cannot hope to do more than just suggest a line of thought, but in every exercise some one must start, and so I beg leave to address you a few words on the above subject.

When a good gardener puts seed into the soil, he takes care that it shall be supplied with whatever experience teaches him is conducive to its development and growth; he does so because he knows that the future plant can be thus modified while still in Nature's earthly womb; indeed, we may say the plant never gets beyond this stage of dependency, as it lacks locomotive power.

We all know how chemistry has been successfully applied to scientific agriculture; and any Hodge looking at a poor crop of wheat in a field will be shrewd enough to surmise that the manuring or tilling had been neglected. He knows full well from what he sees in his own cottage plot that the well-dunged carefully tended portions bear the best crops, and that what grows in this plot is not so readily affected by disease and drought by reason of its more sturdy growth.

Any country schoolboy knows that the poorest apples are on the neglected trees of hedgerows and of neglected grazed orchards, while the fine juicy ones are within the well-kept garden.

Who has not noticed the scraggy, stunted appearance of the calves born of the kine that are turned out to common or forest after they cease to give milk? The future mother-cows lead a hard life, and get but poor sustenance, and their offspring are proportionately undersized and ill-conditioned, and have an ancient, wizened appearance generally.

Similarly, in the human subject, the child of the well-fed, well-worked, cheerful, happy woman, living in a sunlit airy habitation, is at birth the finest specimen of its kind.

On the other hand, what a miserable sight do the new-born babes of our courts and alleys, and of the pampered, tight-laced, high-heeled, lazy, lounging, carriage-possessing women of the higher classes present! The extremes meet; the poor blanched creature, half-starved, overworked, shut up in some close sunless dwelling, brings forth fruit very like that of her pale-faced, over-fed, under-worked, sofa-loving sister of the mansion and of the palace.

And nature is inexorable; look at our bills of infantile mortality if you do not believe it. It is well so; God ordained in His undeviating laws that the fittest should survive, and they do.

Clearly, then, *we may take it for granted that the development of the fruit within the womb can be modified for good and for ill.*

We need not mince the matter; the future human being is made up of four principal factors. First the maternal ovum; secondly, the spermatozoon of the father, which requires, thirdly, a suitable soil for its development and growth. The womb is this suitable soil. These three factors being given, the blood of the mother supplies the fourth.

In the entire plant and animal world, the choice of the seed and soil lies more or less within ken and control, and faulty specimens get a short shrift, while the more fit are allowed to multiply; or in a wild state the weak are crowded out by the strong, and thus the fittest survive.

In our stock-breeding, the bovine and ovine species are well weeded of their faulty and diseased specimens by the butcher. That innocent individual, called the butcher, purchases the rickety or scrofulous calf of the honest farmer, and John Bull enjoys his *Kalb-fleisch* through the Norman medium of veal. Thus nature cares for the survival of the fittest of the bovine species.

With the human species it is very different; faulty specimens of man may not be annihilated for the bettering of the race, and civilized life tends to the protection and fostering of the phy ically faulty, and hence to the deterioration of the race. This is one great reason why civilization tends to the destruction of society through a gradual deterioration of the race by the preservation of the weak from destruction under the reign of law, and by the collateral power of wealth.

In a savage state the weakling goes to the wall; in a civilized state he may be very rich, and of ancient lineage, and then it becomes most important, from the particular standpoint, that he should be married and beget offspring. This ramifies all up and down the various social strata. So in the end the barbarians are strong, and then numerous, and then they break in upon a highly-civilized community, and a reconstruction of society ensues.

It remains to be seen whether science and art will in the future be able to save civilized society from being overwhelmed by savage hordes.

The true source of national greatness is large families of healthy children; these are the only true "fruits of philosophy." Those other "fruits of philosophy" are rotten at the core, and, like all rottenness, lead by the shortest road to annihilation, having here, however, a preliminary stage of bondage and servitude to the seed of the truly philosophically fruitful.

Surely it would be a strange philosophy that came in the mouths of ranting demagogues; *fruit* is the means of reproduction; *Dawn of Destruction* is what they mean.

Mankind is moved to marriage from purely selfish motives; the pairing takes place for almost every reason except for the physical bettering of the race. No doubt it is well so; the production of the most massive members, or of the biggest brains, can hardly be the chief end of man.

Still nature works wisely in making us all, more or less, worshippers of physical beauty and strength; and when the period of motherhood comes nigh, perhaps no greater fear is known than that of ill-formed offspring. It may not be often expressed, but if you could look deep into the sacred secrets of the expectant's heart, you would know that many are the prayers that fly upwards for the great and blessed gift of a *perfect* child.

Is it all right? Is it *perfect?*—is very common y the first question one hears after the newling's *entree au monde.*

To what does all this beauty-worship conduce? To the amelioration of the race. Many an important family has been saved from dying out by a supposedly ignoble *mesalliance.* The British aristocracy is recruited from the ranks of the commoners in more ways than one.

To pretend to inaugurate marriages on racial or scientific grounds is crooked; and although the good old institution known as the family doctor may now and then be asked about the physical desirability of a given projected union, still this is very rare, and when it occurs it usually serves as a cover for other and occult reasons. Therefore, the physicians *role* begins later on. We all know what it usually is.

But to-day I propose directing attention to a subject that has met with but comparatively little notice—certainly with much less than it deserves. I mean the medicinal treatment of the human fruit, while still within the womb, for the cure of hereditary taints and for the prevention of deformity.

My attention was more particularly directed to the subject some six years since in the following manner:

At the end of the year 1874 I was consulted by a gentleman about his children, the youngest of whom had double hare-lip. He had some confidence in Homœopathic treatment, and was desirous of knowing whether there were any means of getting the wound to heal well after the operation for hare-lip that an able surgeon was on the point of undertaking. I recommended the local application of Calendula officinalis as an excellent and well-established vulnerary, especially to clean wounds. The operation took place, the gentleman used the Calendula as directed, and the surgeon, a man of some experience, declared he had never before seen such a rapid healing process or such a nicely-healed surface in any of the cases of hare-lip on which he had operated.

The reputation of Calendula (the common marigold) as a vulnerary is very old, but it survives almost exclusively in the Homœopathic school, in which it is, as you all know, in daily use.

The next older child than the one operated on had, and has, a slight insufficiency of the upper lip; if it were a little worse it would be hare-lip.

Subsequently the gentleman consulted me in regard to his own health, and after the consultation the conversation fell upon his children, upon the excellent result of the operation, and the rapid healing of the wounded parts. Then regret was expressed, especially as the child was a girl, as of course the neatest scar can never constitute a perfect or pretty lip. At the best it is only passable, and not particularly unsightly.

Finally he said, "In case my wife should have another child, what would you expect the next to be like?"

I answered, "That cannot be determined; but taking all the circumstances into consideration, viz., that your first child is perfect, that your second child has only a slight defect in the upper lip, that your third child has double hare-lip, and that your wife was in apparently good health with these, all equally, I should expect the next to have hare-lip also, a little worse than the last, and perhaps even cleft-palate."

He further in uired whether anything could be done to prevent it? My answer was, that I knew of no special experience on the subject at all, but as the body fruit could certainly be affected medicinally, I should think hopefully of properly directed medicinal treatment of the mother during pregnancy. I promised to do my best, and he said he would let me know it any further pregnancy should occur, and place the mother under my treatment.

The subject took hold of my mind, and I often animadverted upon it. Many remedies suggested themselves, and many plans of treatment; the one that found most favor with me was to be based upon specificity of seat or local drug affinity. I reasoned that any drug that would specifically affect the upper lip and palate might act as a stimulus to the part if coursing in the mother's blood, and thus bring about complete union of the bilateral parts. But an insuperable difficulty here presented itself—viz., I knew of no such drug with anything like a strongly-expressed affinity for the part. Such remedies as Kali bichromicum, Aurum, Iodine, Mercury, Natrum muriaticum, Mezereum, Phosphorus, were thought of, but I did not feel the local affinity idea was workable here.

I then thought of tissue affinity or specificity of histological seat, as worked out in its fullest extent of late years by Dr. Schussler, of Oldenburg, in regard to disease. I thought that a formative element of the tissue might be wanting, and thus condition imperfect development. If we grow wheat, we must supply its elements, as manure, to the soil, and if we grow tissue we must supply its elements in the mother's blood which is the food of the fœtus; if the wheat just fail to finish the ear, we conclude formative elements are wanting;, if the absolute concrescence of the bilateral parts of the human fœtus just fails of completion, we may fairly assume that formative elements are lacking. So I thought. And in order to try to find out *what* was likely to be lacking, I went over embryology a little, and I will ask you to go over exactly the same ground as myself presently, by giving a short *resume* of the development of the involved parts first, and then show how, and what remedy I diagnosed.

The surgeon who had operated on the little girl, and also the family accoucheur who assisted at the operation, were also consulted upon the hoped-for possibility of preventive treatment in the then future; but these gentlemen laughed at the idea, and said the only thing for it was operation, prevention being out of the question.

But we may reflect upon the fact that it is not at all an uncommon thing in our hospitals, and occasionally in general practice, to treat a pregnant person suffering from syphilis very actively with Mercury, and the results are on the whole very encouraging indeed; still, as far as I am aware, it is seldom that any physician attempts the intra-uterine treatment of any other complaint, and even here the *idea* has generally been to treat the *mother* only, or principally.

In thinking the matter over, and endeavouring to find some sound reason to guide me in the to-be-attempted preventive treatment of hare-lip, I was encouraged to hope for a good result from the recorded experience of a few Homœopathic obstetricians who tell us of the successful medicinal treatment of the uterus and of he expectant mother herself; for it seemed no great difficulty, theoretically, to modify the development of the fœtus, which grows in the uterus and is fed with the blood of the mother, seeing that both the mother's blood and uterus can, demonstrably, be modified therapeutically.

Now, although I felt the idea of trying to prevent hare-lip with the help of *specificity of seat* in the ordinary Homœopathic sense unworkable, still this lay in the nature of the case rather than in the nature of the thing generally. Thus in those liable to beget offspring with defects or deformities, or displacements of organs, or parts to which we have approved remedies with specific affinities for such organs or parts, we might, and undoubtedly should, find it of eminent service, and also of the careful application of the Homœopathic law of similars; also of the tripartite pathology of Hahnemann; and of the constitutional states of Grauvogl, and perhaps, even of the *Remedia universalia* of Rademacher.[1]

But to return, let us examine the embryology of the parts involved in hare-lip and cleft-palate.

Biologists tell us that the face is originally formed of a middle portion proceeding from the forehead, or frontal process, and of a lateral portion on each side, derived from the superior extremity of the first visceral arch. These parts are at first separate.

The lateral and the inferior parts, destined to form the superior and inferior maxillary apparatus, are both derived from the first visceral arch, in which an angular bend appears; the part above this bend being converted into the superior maxillary mass, and that below it into the inferior maxillary apparatus.

The superior maxillary mass, in its growth, approaches the frontal process, and unites with it; a cavity being left between that process and the two superior maxillary masses, which becomes the nasal cavity. By the union of the superior maxillary masses (the superior maxilla and palate bone) of opposite sides beneath this cavity, the separation of the nose from the mouth by the palate is effected.

1 *Remedium universale* is not a would-be panacea or cure-all, but one that hypothetically affects the universe of the microcosm, *i. e.*, not an organ.

The mode of development of the face affords an explanation of the abnormal cleft palate, and the congenital cleft between the upper maxillary and the intermaxillary bones and of those congenital fissures which pass between the intermaxillary and upper jaw, as far upwards as the orbital cavity. Congenital clefts of this kind are thus the *results of an arrest of development occurring during the primitive conditions of the parts.*

We may, therefore, infer that cleft-palate is due to lack of a due supply of formative material; the superior maxillary masses ossify indeed, but fail to unite in the median lines. If so it will follow that if the requisite amount of formative matter be supplied soon enough to the maternal blood, it will be given off to the fœtus, and tissued osseous union will take place, and deformity will be prevented.

But the skeleton may unite in the middle, and yet the soft parts fail to do so; and when this occurs with those of the superior maxilla, the deformity known as hare-lip is the result.

We may regard the basis of the upper lip structure as already differentiated into connective tissue, which is indeed the stroma of the whole body, and of all its organs. When, therefore, the soft parts fail to unite in the median line of the upper lip, and we get the ugly defect known as hare-lip, we may conclude that the development became arrested from a lack of one of its constituents *in developmental or functional power.*

All things considered, I concluded it was, in this case, *lack of lime-life.*

Then the next point was—which salt of lime? Here the psoric constitution of the mother pointed to Sulphur.

My conception was not that there was an actual lack of lime as such, but rather a lack of assimilative or developmental power of the lime-function in the sense of Moleschott and of Schussler, and that struma or psora (= morbid x) was the hindering agent.

I therefore decided on Calcarea sulphurica, and believing it was *quality* that was required, and *not quantity*, I determined on the sixth centesimal trituration.

This is how I diagnosed, theoretically, a remedy for *this case* of presumptive defective formation, and this remedy I made up my mind to give if the lady should come under my care.

A little time elapsed, and the husband appeared to inform me that his wife was believed to be *enceinte.* Calcarea sulphurica, 6th trituration, one grain night and morning, was prescribed. The lady continued to take it till the end of the seventh month of pregnancy, and during the last two months she took Lithium carbonicum, and at full term *she gave birth to a healthy and perfect child.*

In due course a *second* pregnancy took place. The same course of treatment was adopted, and with the same happy result—viz., *a perfect child.*

Since this time I have kept the subject of the intra-uterine medicinal treatment of the human fœtus before my mind; but my experience here has since been for the purpose of preventing, respectively eradicating, constitutional taints and hereditary proclivities. Cases other than those two, for the prevention of defect or deformity, have not hitherto come under my observation.

But this further experience of mine I will refer to again, as an interesting paper, published in the *Practitioner* for December, 1878, by Dr. Thomas P. Tuckey, of County Cork, Ireland, here claims attention. Dr. Tuckey is evidently an original thinker. This paper is entitled, "On the Preventive Treatment of Cleft-palate and Hare-lip, and some further Remarks on the Relation of the Ovaries to the Sex of the child."

Our author tells us that his attention was directed some years ago to the remarkable success which has attended the Dublin Zoological Society in the breeding of lions, and the great immunity which animals born in their gardens, in the Phœnix Gardens, enjoy from various disorders and deformities to which the lion bred in a state of subjection is liable. The most remarkable of these diseases is cleft-palate, which lions in a captive state are very apt to have. Dr. Tuekey, believes it was the Rev. Professor Haughton, when speaking before some public assembly, who drew attention to this fact and stated that it was his opinion that the cause ot the lions in the Dublin Gardens being born so unblemished was giving the mothers bones which they could crush. This faet very much impressed Dr. Tuekey, and as he happened to have under his observation a family of several children who were all, both male and female, subject to hare-lips, several of which cases were complicated with cleft-palate, he determined to speak to the mother, who was in poor circumstances, and ask her to let him know the next time she was in the family-way, that he might give her a medicine which would prevent her next child having the same deformity as the others. The poor woman was heart-broken, taking her children here and there to be operated upon, and quite jumped at the idea, and promised faithfully to come and report herself the moment she bel eved herself to be *enceinte.*

This is the woman's family history:

Mrs. H., aged thirty-five, mother of six children. Every one of her children have had hare-lips, two have also had cleft-palate. The disease appeared not to be hereditary, and she could not call to mind any of her family, or of her husband's family, who have had hare-lips. Is a fine strong woman, but has fearfully crooked eyes; no other deformity. Has always had good health. Her husband, small, but strong and healthy, never has had any diseases while she has been married to him. He and she have both lived all their lives in the country. He is sober, and has always been so. Her first child had simple hare-lip; no cleft in palate; does not remember getting any frights when carrying her hildren.

A pregnancy occurred; Mrs. H. presented herself, and the doctor prescribed the following mixture:

℞ Calcis phos. ʒj. grs. 20.
Calcis carb. ʒj.
Bicarb. magnes.
Chlorid. sodii.
Sodæ. phosph. a a ℈ ss. M.

To be added to an 8 oz. mixture composed of Gelatine, Gum arabic, Syrup of ginger, and Cinnamon water; 1 drachm three times daily.

As clefts in the palate and lip are said to be due to arrest of development prior to the end of the third month, Mrs. H. was at once put on this mixture, which is intended to represent a very rough analysis of the constituents of bone. In any future cases Dr. T. thinks he would grind up the bones of the head of some animal, and give some of the powder instead of the above elaborately constructed mixture.

The essential parts of this mixture are clearly the Lime, Phosphorus, and Magnesia. The little poly-pharmaceutical performance of adding Gelatine, Gum arabic, Syrup of ginger, and Cinnamon water is not a little amusing.

But to return. The woman took the mixture regularly until the fourth month; she went her full time, and was delivered of a girl, without a trace of deformity about her lips or palate; the child was healthy and strong.

Hearing of this case, a Mrs. L. came to seek Dr. Tuckey's advice. She was the mother of eight children, most of whom had cleft-palate and hare-lips; in four of them the hare-lip was double, and more shocking objects of deformity he had never seen. One boy was perfectly repulsive. The woman believed herself pregnant, and was at once put on the mixture. She went her full time, bore a girl without hare-lip, indeed, *but who evidently had had one in utero*, for the lip, though united, was united *crookedly*, and one side was puckered up, as if by a slight and narrow burn.

This is, truly, a most remarkable and interesting case.

I must demur to the statement that the arrest of development occurring before a certain period necessarily involves the conclusion that treatment in the latter months of gestation would be useless. This is a pure assumption, and based on normal observations. Here we have to do with arrested and *therefore retarded* growth, and hence the nutritional or medicinal treatment should not only be begun early, but continued to the end; and one begun late would still be hopeful of obtaining amelioration, if not of complete normality.

Again, there is an objection to the use of the bone, simply as the lips have not the same constituents as the bones, and in the same proportions; so if we are to give pulverized heads we must give the lips too.

But we, happily, need neither one nor the other; neither do we need any bulky, cunningly-devised mixture, with nasty or nice additions, to mystify, and obscure, and render our own observations open to objections.

Pure clinical experiment must be with one remedy at a time to be conclusive.

Thus, I may object to Dr. Tuckey's proposition that the Phosphates did the work in his cases, on the ground that the tincture of ginger acted as a stomachic, and strengthened his patient's digestions, so that they assimilated more food, and *thus* were the defects prevented. Another might attribute it to the Gelatine; a third to the Alcohol, a fourth to the Cinnamon.

Then this polypharmacy prevents individualizing, which is the soul of all true progress in scientific medicine.

I was once struck with the extreme beauty of a lady's children, both parents being rather plain, and found that she had been in the habit of using a mixture of Phosphorus, Iron, and sherry during gestation to keep her strength up. Her own health was seriously injured by it.

I think it will be conceded that it is at least highly probable that the preventive treatment of congenital deformities and defects may be undertaken with good chances of success, and I venture to submit that this corner of the field of practical medicine is well worthy the attention and skill of all physicians, and also of all well-wishers of the race, lay as well as medical.

It will be of surpassing interest to the individuals and families more immediately interested, through having undesirable family proclivities.

There is here great scope for the tissue remedies, especially when dynamized, as it is likely to be qualitatively changed nutritive building material that is required.

No doubt the various cases of congenital defect and deformity differ essentially in their natures, and will require accordingly different remedial or preventive treatment.

This immense field lies fallow ready for the tilling talents of willing workers.

As soon as this is undertaken, facts will multiply, and reliable data will be at hand to guide us.

To draw a line of demarcation between the nutritional and medicinal treatment is not now possible. Undoubtedly some cases will require nutritional treatment solely; others will require medicinal treatment directed to the mother's constitutional crasis; in others, again, a debilitated generative sphere may claim attention. Or a presumable taint in the marital product may call for the principal intra-uterine therapeutic endeavours.

Here I may narrate the following observation. A lady patient of mine was extremely fond of liver, during one of her pregnancies; at least once a week she would partake copiously of it—pregnancy fads are as old as the world. This lady was delivered of a very fine *child that had extensive pigmentation of the forehead*, such as we are wont to see in some ladies during gestation. This brown discoloration gradually disappeared from the baby's forehead in about four weeks. The mother's skin was also in parts very deeply pigmented, but not the forehead.

Hitherto we have referred more particularly to the preventive nutritional and medicinal treatment of defects and deformities; it has, we opine, a certain future.

Perhaps it will now be profitable to consider the subject of disease from the same standpoint.

To start with, we may not do amiss to realize the fact that we get, so to speak, a capital leverage for our therapeutical work, inasmuch as we have a number of months in which to accomplish it. We know from daily experience that numerous diseases can be cured by a *course of treatment* spread over a considerable period of time, but which cannot be modified to any great extent with any *one* given remedy.

The various remedies follow one another like steps in a staircase, and they are all needful to reach the top.

Then we have the most favorable physical conditions. Our fœtal patients are not exposed to change of temperature, but have a constant temperature in the best possible medium, and they are pretty sure to take their physic regularly.

Ever since my attention was arrested, as before stated, by the observations of hare-lip, I have sought opportunities of testing the truth of this theory—that the body fruit, while still within the womb, can be nutritionally and medicinally modified at will. Further cases of deformity have not presented themselves, but in general practice I have had some opportunities of observing the beneficial effects of the medicinal treatment of pregnant women for the prevention of various to-be-expected morbid states.

Thus, a lady patient of mine has a good many moles and warts on her person, and her husband a great number of warts, some very unsightly, on his. Considering the frequent observations that warts will, at a more advanced period of life, take on increased action, hypertrophy, and become epitheliomatous, their presence in an individual is not only æsthetically undesirable, but may become the source of positive danger to life; at any rate, they are ugly things at the best. Moreover, both of them are rheumatic and constitutionally strumous. This lady has passed through four pregnancies under my observation and professional care, and during each one I subjected her to a course of treatment with the most happy results. The four children were born with unblemished skins—wartless, moleless, and spotlessly pure.

It may be objected that the treatment had nothing to do

with this purity of skin, as the interesting babes might have been equally unblemished, without any treatment at all. Of course, I cannot *prove* the contrary, still—

> "Like genders like, potatoes tatoes breed,
> Uncostly ca bage springs from cabbage seed."

My belief is, and it is based on observation, that those four children would in all probability have all been born with unsightly warts on various parts of their persons had the mother not been treated to prevent it.

The course of treatment followed was in this wise—*a peu prés.*

Sulphur, generally in the sixth, twelfth, or thirtieth dilution (by preference the last-named), was given as the most certain anti-psoric. This was granted time to act, and then followed Thuja occidentalis as *the* anti-sycotic *par excellence.* Lest any specific taint lay in its history, Mercurius was given. The lady's teeth are very carious, and hence Acidum fluoricum was given for a while; the children have thus far sound toothie-peggies, and teethed normally and without any mediævally superstitious gum-lancing.

Apropos of gum-lancing, if those who still adhere to this barbarous practice would just work up the indications of Aconite, Belladonna, Ferrum phos., Kreasote, Calcarea carb., Calcarea fluorica, Silicea, Phosphorus, and the like, they would soon have, as I have, a *very* rusty lancet, and a very grateful heart, that they no longer need to pain the poor bairns and constitute themselves dreaded objects. Moreover, they would soon satisfy themselves, after a little careful observation, that the gums are not the offending parts, but the unfinished, abnormally constituted *teeth*, and a morbid something lying behind and beyond in the constitutional crasis. *Sapientibus sat.*

A lady, mother of several (five) children, was under my

treatment for a chronic internal skin affection; her husband had formerly been successfully treated by me, for psoriasis of lower extremities, with Arsenicum.

The last baby I had treated for eczema while still at the breast, and when it was vaccinated the arm became very seriously inflamed, and the object of anxious care and medicinal treatment. All the five children had had, I was informed something wrong with the skin, and every scratch with them festered.

The sixth pregnancy occurred, and I treated the lady during the greater portion of it. The principal remedies used were Psorinum 30, Sulphur 30, Calc. sulph. 6, and Juglans cinerea 1.

The child came in due course; everything was normal, and the little mannikin was the finest of the lot, and remained for two years with a pure skin, and the vaccination caused no inconvenience. All the other children had had cutaneous affections before they were a year old, and some of them proved altogether intractable.

The child passed from my observation then, but I have heard that it now has "something on its arm," but what I do not know. Supposing it to be a cutaneous affection, the result of the preventive treatment would be that it remained free for the first two years of its life; and moreover, it is by far the finest and handsomest of the six children.

Of course I cannot *prove* that it would have been otherwise if the mother had had no treatment at all.

It was once my duty to treat a conjugal pair, each for the morbus gallicus, that admittedly was a marital acquisition. A pregnancy occurred while only too many unmistakable symyptoms were objects of treatment. During almost the whole of the pregnancy the lady was persistently treated with Mercurius, Aurum, Stillingia sylvatica, and the like, with an occasional pause. The usual term of utero-gestation resulted in the birth of an apparently perfectly healthy spotless child, and, as long as I observed it, it remained so.

No doubt other practitioners are in the habit of treating pregnant women for various ailments, and will be able, from longer experience and greater opportunities than mine, to give more striking examples of its efficacy in regard to the mothers, and perhaps also *quo ad* the offspring.

Having thus gone rapidly over the subject of the prevention of defect, deformity, and diseases by the intra-uterine medicinal and nutritional treatment of the pregnant person during gestation, it only remains for me to apologize for the meagreness of the practical suggestions I am able to offer in the few minutes allotted to me for this paper, and to express a hope that you will freely add hereto in the discussion which is to follow, so that it may be said that I merely give out the text and you, gentlemen, preach the sermon.

[Before reading this paper of Dr. Burnett my attention was called to the possible relations of cleft-palate in the child and gastric disorders of the mother.

I was called one day last fall to see a mother who had been del vered of an eight month's child about six weeks before. She was suffering severely with gastralgia. I found the case to be one of gastric catarrh and treated her accordingly with the best results. The child was a small one and was put upon milk as it had difficulty of nursing from the partial cleft in the palate, besides the mother had only a little milk and that I judged not of the best quality.

The general symptoms of this case recalled a similar one

that I had treated about ten years before. In this instance the child had not only complete cleft palate, but also double hare-lip. The gastric catarrh of the mother was cured and a subsequent child was born perfect. It might be of interest to add that the first mother had morbus coxarius when young, and that the second mother was of a tubercular diathesis—the disease being now apparently held in check by Homœopathic remedies.

That persistent gastric disorders in the early months of pregnancy must seriously interfere with the nutrition of the child is doubtless true, but whether gastric catarrh alone is responsible for congenital malformations or defects, except in a general way, is a problem worthy of farther attention.]